ATRIAL FIBRILLATION THERAPY

Integrative Therapies For Heart Rhythm Harmony

Find Freedom From Atrial Fibrillation With Integrative Therapies Promoting Heart Rhythm Harmony And Cardiovascular Health

JAMES JOSEPH

CHAPTER ONE

Introduction

Atrial fibrillation (AFib) is a common cardiac rhythm disease marked by irregular and typically fast heartbeats. When the heart's upper chambers (atria) quiver instead of contracting regularly, blood flow might be disrupted, possibly leading to issues such as blood clots, stroke, or heart failure.

While traditional treatments for AFib exist, there is a growing acknowledgment of the advantages of integrative therapies, which emphasize the significance of holistic methods that address not just the physical symptoms but also the underlying causes of the disorder.

Understanding atrial fibrillation

Atrial fibrillation is a complicated cardiac disease that alters the heart's natural rhythm. Individuals with AFib suffer erratic and disorganized electrical impulses rather than synchronized contractions, which effectively pump blood. This erratic pulse may lead to poor blood circulation, which raises the chance of blood clots developing in the atrium. When these clots go to the brain, they may cause a stroke, therefore AFib is a severe medical worry.

AFib has a variety of causes, including aging, high blood pressure, cardiac disease, heavy alcohol intake, and other chronic illnesses. Understanding the underlying causes of atrial fibrillation is critical for successful management and therapy.

Conventional Treatments: Pros and Cons

Conventional AFib therapies try to restore normal cardiac rhythm, manage heart rate, and avoid problems. Common medical therapies include anti-arrhythmic medicines, blood thinners to avoid clots, and procedures such as cardioversion or catheter ablation.

While these medicines may help manage AFib, they are not without disadvantages. Anti-arrhythmic drugs may have adverse effects, and their long-term effectiveness may be restricted due to their effects on other organs. Blood thinners, although necessary for avoiding strokes, have their own set of drawbacks, including an increased chance of bleeding. While catheter ablation is frequently effective, it may contain certain hazards and may not be appropriate for everyone.

Individuals with AFib must work closely with their healthcare professionals to assess the advantages and dangers of standard therapies and choose the best method for their circumstances.

The Role of Integrative Therapies

Integrative treatments take a holistic approach to healthcare, recognizing the interdependence of the mind, body, and spirit. Integrative therapies for AFib attempt to supplement traditional treatments by addressing lifestyle variables, boosting general well-being, and minimizing the influence of stress on the cardiovascular system.

Acupuncture, yoga, massage, and other techniques have shown potential in improving heart health and alleviating AFib symptoms. Integrating integrative treatments into a complete treatment plan may improve the efficacy of traditional medical procedures while also improving an individual's overall quality of life.

CHAPTER TWO

Mind-Body Connection: Stress Reduction Techniques.

Stress is a recognized cause of AFib episodes and may worsen the illness in people who are already afflicted. Therefore, reducing stress is a vital component of AFib management. Stress reduction approaches based on the mind-body link have received attention for their potential advantages in controlling AFib.

Meditation and mindfulness may help people build a feeling of calm and minimize their physiological reactions to stress. Deep breathing techniques, guided visualization, and progressive muscle relaxation are all strategies that may be used in everyday life to promote relaxation and lessen the effects of stress on the cardiovascular system.

Yoga, which combines physical postures, breathwork, and meditation, has shown promise in improving heart health and may be especially good for those who have AFib. Individuals should check with their healthcare practitioners before beginning new fitness programs, particularly if they have pre-existing cardiovascular issues.

Individuals with AFib may enjoy a decrease in the frequency and severity of episodes by managing stress with these mind-body connection approaches, resulting in greater overall heart health.

Balancing Nutrition for Heart Health

Diet is essential for heart health, and for those with AFib, eating a heart-healthy diet is especially vital. A well-balanced diet may improve cardiovascular health, aid with weight management, and lower the risk of other diseases that might cause AFib.

A heart-healthy diet often consists of nutrient-dense foods including fruits, vegetables, whole grains, lean meats, and healthy fats. Limiting processed meals, salt, and saturated fats may help improve cardiovascular health.

Certain dietary concerns may be unique to those with AFib. For example, various meals and drinks, including caffeine and alcohol, might cause AFib episodes in some individuals. Understanding personal triggers and making suitable dietary changes might help manage AFib symptoms.

To summarize, complete care of AFib entails recognizing the problem, weighing the pros and drawbacks of traditional medications, combining integrative therapies, treating the mind-body link via stress reduction strategies, and adopting a heart-healthy diet. Individuals who take a holistic approach to AFib treatment may improve their entire well-being and quality of life while successfully managing the problems associated with this cardiovascular ailment. Consult a healthcare expert for individualized advice and assistance targeted to your specific health requirements.

Finding the right balance between exercise and atrial fibrillation

Atrial Fibrillation (AFib) is a common cardiac rhythm disease in which the atria beat irregularly and rapidly. It may cause a variety of consequences, including a higher risk of stroke and heart failure. While exercise is usually helpful to heart health, people with AFib often ask what the correct balance is between being active and avoiding triggers for their illness.

Herbal Treatments and Supplements for Heart Rhythm Stability

In addition to standard medical therapies, some people use herbal remedies and supplements to control AFib and increase cardiac rhythm stability. It is critical to explore these alternatives carefully and under the supervision of healthcare specialists.

Certain plants, such as hawthorn, motherwort, and valerian, have long been linked to cardiovascular health. However, their efficacy in treating AFib has not been proven, and their interaction with prescription drugs must be carefully evaluated. Magnesium and omega-3 fatty acid supplements are also known to have heart-healthy properties. However, further study is needed to determine their influence on AFib.

Before adopting herbal therapies or supplements into an AFib management strategy, patients should check with their healthcare practitioners to establish their safety and efficacy. It is important to understand that natural does not necessarily imply safety and interactions with prescription pharmaceuticals may have unforeseen results.

CHAPTER THREE

Acupuncture and Traditional Chinese Medicine Approaches

Acupuncture, a major component of Traditional Chinese Medicine (TCM), is the insertion of tiny needles into particular spots on the body. Some AFib patients see acupuncture as an alternative or supplemental therapy to traditional therapies.

TCM sees the body as an interrelated system that requires balance for optimal health. Acupuncture strives to restore balance and stimulate the flow of vital energy, or qi, throughout the body. While there is minimal scientific data on the efficacy of acupuncture for AFib, some research shows that it may help general cardiovascular health and reduce stress.

Individuals seeking acupuncture for AFib should visit their doctors. Acupuncture is usually regarded safe when conducted by skilled practitioners, although it must be used in conjunction with conventional therapies rather than in place of them.

Yoga and meditation: cultivating inner calm

Yoga and meditation have grown in popularity as holistic techniques to treat a variety of health ailments, including cardiovascular diseases such as AFib. These practices focus on the mind-body link, encouraging relaxation, stress reduction, and general well-being.

Yoga for AFib

Yoga, with its focus on gentle movements, regulated breathing, and meditation, may be beneficial for those with AFib. Certain yoga postures and sequences may be modified to meet the specific demands and limits of people who have cardiac rhythm issues. However, it is critical to approach yoga with care and choose teachers who have prior experience dealing with people who have cardiovascular issues.

Individuals with AFib should visit their healthcare practitioners before beginning a yoga practice to verify that certain postures or activities will not aggravate their condition. Yoga should be introduced gently, and any pain or unpleasant reactions should be treated immediately with medical advice.

Meditation techniques

Meditation, such as mindfulness meditation and guided imagery, may be beneficial for stress management and emotional well-being. Stress is a recognized cause of AFib episodes, and developing inner peace via meditation may help minimize their frequency and severity.

Meditation may improve heart health by reducing blood pressure and encouraging calm. However, it is critical to understand that meditation is a supplement to and should not replace recommended medical therapies.

Finding Personalized Solutions

Management of AFib is very customized, and what works for one person may not work for others. Individuals with AFib should collaborate closely with their healthcare professionals to build a thorough and tailored treatment strategy.

While researching complementary and alternative treatments such as herbal remedies, acupuncture, yoga, and meditation, it is critical to keep open contact with medical specialists. These techniques should be seen as part of a comprehensive plan that complements rather than replaces traditional therapies.

Individuals dealing with AFib must find a careful balance between standard medical therapies and other methods. Exercise is an important component of heart health, but finding the proper balance is critical for people with AFib. Herbal medicines, acupuncture, yoga, and meditation give additional options for assistance, but their efficacy and safety must be carefully considered and discussed with healthcare experts.

Finally, the integration of these complementary treatments should be treated from a holistic perspective, acknowledging the interconnectedness of the mind and body. Individuals with AFib may create a complete plan that addresses both the physical and emotional components of their disease, to live a balanced and well-managed lifestyle.

CHAPTER FOUR

Biofeedback and Heart Coherence Techniques

Biofeedback and cardiac coherence techniques have developed as potential methods for controlling a variety of cardiovascular diseases, including atrial fibrillation (AF). These approaches make use of the link between the mind and the body, enabling people to develop greater control over physiological systems. These strategies are useful for preventing and managing AF, a common cardiac arrhythmia characterized by irregular heartbeats.

The concept of biofeedback and heart coherence

Biofeedback is the real-time monitoring of physiological characteristics such as heart rate, blood pressure, and muscular tension to give people instant information about their physical functioning. In contrast, cardiac coherence refers to a condition of physiological synchronization in which heart rate variability becomes more orderly and rhythmic. Heart coherence is linked to lower stress, higher emotional well-being, and better cardiovascular health.

In the context of AF, biofeedback and cardiac coherence approaches try to modify the autonomic nerve system, which is responsible for regulating heart function. These strategies enable people to favorably impact their heart rhythm by teaching them to develop coherence using methods such as guided breathing exercises and mindfulness.

The impact of sleep on atrial fibrillation

Sleep is essential for cardiovascular health, and irregular sleep patterns have been related to an increased risk of developing atrial fibrillation. Poor sleep quality, poor sleep length, and disorders such as sleep apnea may all contribute to the development and progression of AF. Understanding and resolving sleep-related issues are critical components of a comprehensive strategy for managing atrial fibrillation.

Both biofeedback and heart coherence approaches may help improve sleep quality. These techniques promote relaxation, reduce tension, and encourage mental and physiological coherence, all of which lead to improved sleep hygiene. Integrating these strategies into a comprehensive AF treatment strategy acknowledges the link between sleep and cardiovascular health.

Managing atrial fibrillation in dally llfe

Living with atrial fibrillation requires a proactive and comprehensive strategy for managing symptoms and improving overall well-being. Individuals with AF need lifestyle changes, such as stress management and relaxation strategies, in addition to medicinal therapies.

Biofeedback and heart coherence methods are useful tools for treating atrial fibrillation in everyday life. Guided imagery, deep breathing exercises, and mindfulness meditation may all help to reduce stress, regulate emotions, and promote heart coherence. These strategies enable people to take an active part in their health, supplementing medical therapies and instilling a feeling of control over their condition.

CHAPTER FIVE

Personalized Treatment Plans:

Understanding Your Options

Given the variable nature of atrial fibrillation and the distinct aspects of each person's health profile, tailored treatment regimens are required. Biofeedback and cardiac coherence methods help to individualize therapy by providing adaptive tools that may be adapted to each patient's unique requirements and preferences.

Individuals with atrial fibrillation may research and incorporate biofeedback and heart coherence approaches into their tailored treatment programs by working with healthcare providers.

This collaborative approach encourages patients to actively engage in their treatment, instilling a feeling of ownership and dedication to managing their disease.

Case Studies: Success Stories in Atrial Fibrillation Freedom

Real-life experiences and success stories demonstrate the effectiveness of biofeedback and heart coherence approaches in controlling atrial fibrillation.

Case studies show how people have integrated these techniques into their everyday lives, resulting in better symptoms, a higher quality of life, and, in some instances, a decrease in the frequency of atrial fibrillation episodes.

For example, a case study may depict a person who, in addition to medical therapies, engaged in frequent biofeedback sessions and heart coherence activities. Consistent administration resulted in a significant reduction in stress levels, enhanced emotional well-being, and a subjective decrease in the intensity and frequency of atrial fibrillation episodes. Such success examples demonstrate the value of these strategies as part of a comprehensive strategy for AF management.

In the treatment of atrial fibrillation, biofeedback, and cardiac coherence methods provide a comprehensive and individualized approach that goes beyond typical medical therapies. These activities encourage people to actively participate in their well-being by giving tools for stress reduction, emotional balance, and increased heart coherence.

Recognizing the interconnection of physiological and psychological components allows patients to manage the intricacies of atrial fibrillation with a thorough and individualized treatment strategy. Success stories in atrial fibrillation freedom demonstrate the possibility of these strategies to enhance symptoms and general quality of life. As our awareness of the mind-body link grows, biofeedback and cardiac coherence methods remain at the forefront of novel approaches to cardiovascular health, providing hope and empowerment to patients suffering from atrial fibrillation.

In the quest for long-term well-being, people often seek holistic treatments that address several elements of their health. One such way is to work with healthcare specialists to identify possible hazards and take appropriate safeguards, particularly when it comes to heart rhythm harmony.

Potential Risks and Precautions

Maintaining cardiac rhythm harmony is critical for general health since any interruption might result in major health complications. Before beginning on a holistic route to long-term health, it is important to be informed of the hazards. Heart rhythm problems, commonly known as arrhythmias, may be caused by a variety of factors, including genetics, lifestyle, and underlying medical illnesses.

When pursuing holistic techniques, individuals should proceed with care and keep pre-existing health issues in mind. For example, some herbal supplements or alternative treatments may interfere with heart-related drugs. It is important to speak with healthcare specialists before introducing new items into one's wellness regimen to ensure that there are no negative side effects or contraindications.

CHAPTER SIX
Collaboration with Healthcare Professionals

Collaboration with healthcare providers is an essential component of holistic well-being. A holistic approach mixes alternative therapies with traditional medicine, recognizing that each plays an important part in sustaining a person's entire health.

Healthcare specialists such as cardiologists, dietitians, and holistic practitioners may collaborate to develop a complete wellness strategy. This partnership guarantees that all facets of an individual's health are evaluated, allowing for a more personalized approach that meets unique needs and concerns. Regular check-ups and discussions with healthcare experts are vital for tracking success and making modifications to the wellness plan as required.

Individuals seeking a comprehensive approach to heart rhythm harmony should communicate their aspirations with their healthcare team. Open communication allows specialists to give advice, assess possible dangers, and provide individualized recommendations based on a person's specific health profile.

A holistic approach to long-term wellness

A holistic approach to long-term well-being addresses the physical, mental, and emotional elements of health. It goes beyond just treating symptoms, aiming to uncover and address the underlying causes of imbalance. This technique combines a variety of lifestyle variables and actions to promote heart rhythm harmony.

1. Nutrition: Eating a heart-healthy diet rich in fruits, vegetables, whole grains, and lean meats is essential. Nutrient-dense meals provide the body with important vitamins and minerals, which promote overall cardiovascular health.

2. Physical Activity: Regular exercise is essential for preserving heart rhythm harmony. Activities such as brisk walking, swimming, and yoga improve cardiovascular fitness and lower the incidence of arrhythmias.

3. Stress Management: Chronic stress may have a harmful influence on heart health. To improve emotional well-being, holistic wellness emphasizes stress reduction strategies such as meditation, deep breathing exercises, and mindfulness practices.

4. Quality Sleep: Inadequate sleep may disturb the body's normal rhythms, especially the heart rate. Establishing appropriate sleep patterns improves

overall heart health and promotes a holistic approach to well-being.

5. Holistic therapies include acupuncture, massage, and biofeedback, which may supplement traditional therapy for cardiac rhythm abnormalities. These treatments aim to restore the body's balance and equilibrium.

Conclusion: Embracing Heart-Rhythm Harmony

Finally, achieving heart rhythm harmony requires a comprehensive and holistic strategy that takes into account both traditional and alternative approaches. Recognizing possible dangers and adopting essential safeguards, particularly while working with healthcare providers, enables a well-rounded and tailored wellness journey.

A harmonic heart rhythm is more than just the absence of problems; it is a condition of optimum functioning and balance. Individuals may strive toward and maintain heart rhythm harmony by including diet, physical exercise, stress management, adequate sleep, and holistic treatments in their daily routines.

The route to long-term well-being is continual and dynamic. Regular evaluations, changes, and consultation with healthcare specialists are the core of a comprehensive strategy. Finally, the objective is not only to avoid sickness but to cultivate a happy and balanced existence in which heart rhythm harmony is a natural reflection of total health.

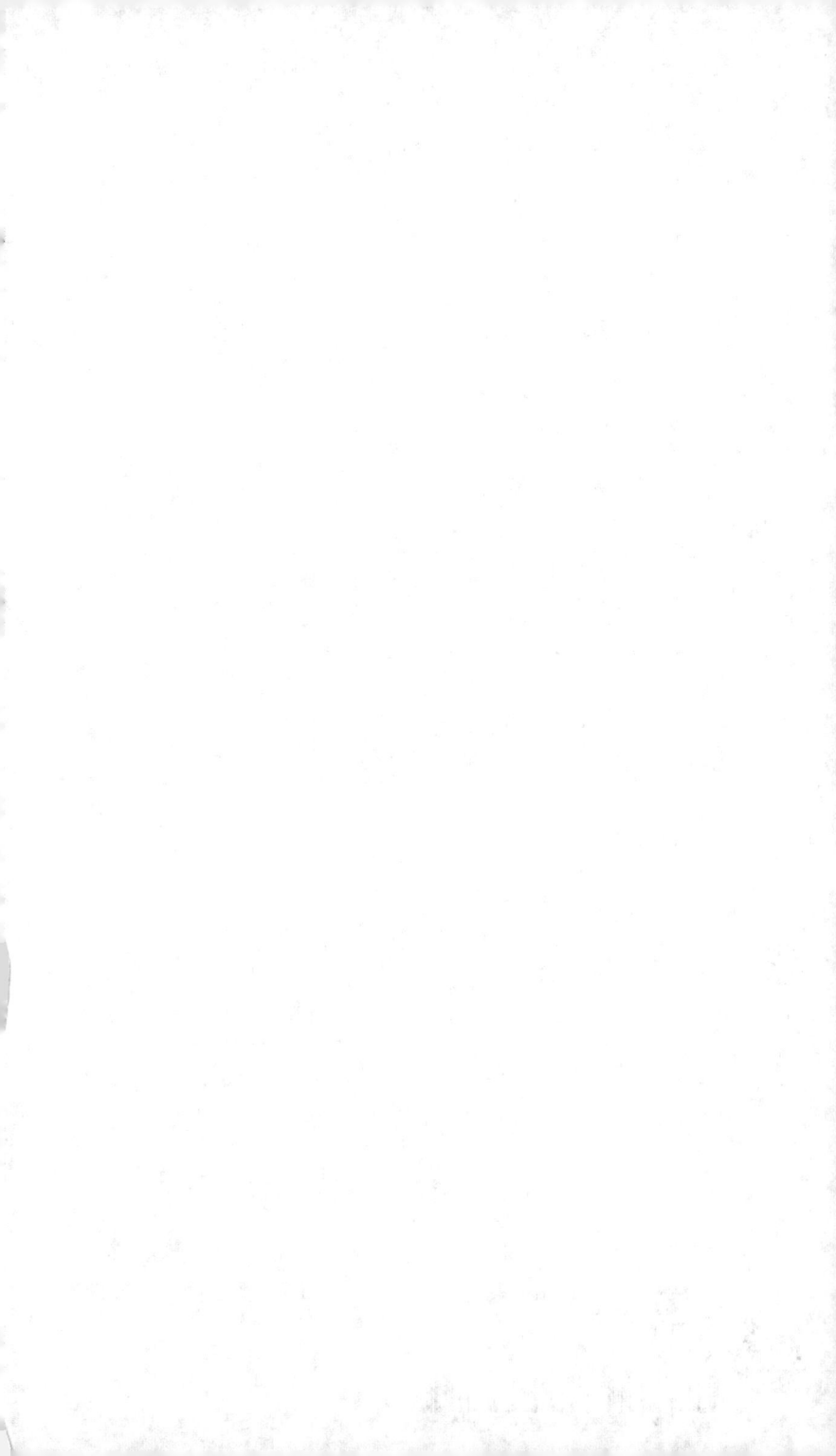